The Easy Weight Loss Challenge: 30 Days to a New You

karthikeya muthu and Maximus

Published by K studio, 2024.

While every precaution has been taken in the preparation of this book, the publisher assumes no responsibility for errors or omissions, or for damages resulting from the use of the information contained herein.

THE EASY WEIGHT LOSS CHALLENGE: 30 DAYS TO A NEW YOU

First edition. December 3, 2024.

Written by karthikeya muthu and Maximus.

Introduction

Have you ever looked in the mirror and felt dissatisfied with what you saw? Do you find yourself constantly battling with the scale, trying fad diets, or feeling overwhelmed by the thought of transforming your body? If so, you're not alone. Millions of people worldwide struggle with their weight, often feeling trapped in a cycle of frustration and disappointment. But what if I told you that in just 30 days, you could kickstart a journey to a healthier, happier you? Welcome to "The Easy Weight Loss Challenge: 30 Days to a New You," a comprehensive guide that will revolutionize your approach to weight loss and empower you to take control of your health and well-being.

In today's fast-paced world, where convenience foods and sedentary lifestyles have become the norm, maintaining a healthy weight has become increasingly challenging. The statistics are staggering: obesity rates continue to climb, and weight-related health issues are on the rise. However, amidst this troubling trend, there's hope. The solution lies not in extreme measures or quick fixes, but in sustainable, science-backed strategies that can be easily integrated into your daily life. This book is your roadmap to achieving lasting weight loss success, offering a structured 30-day program that combines nutrition, exercise, and lifestyle modifications to help you shed pounds and keep them off for good.

What sets "The Easy Weight Loss Challenge" apart from other weight loss books is its holistic, practical approach. Rather than promoting restrictive diets or grueling workout regimens, this book focuses on making small, manageable changes that add up to significant results. Drawing from the latest research in nutrition, exercise science, and behavioral psychology, we've distilled the most effective weight loss strategies into a user-friendly program that anyone can follow. Whether you're a busy professional, a stay-at-home parent, or someone who's tried and failed at weight loss before, this book is designed to meet you where you are and guide you to where you want to be.

Throughout the pages of this book, you'll discover several key themes that form the foundation of successful weight loss. First and foremost is the concept of balance. We'll explore how to create a balanced approach to nutrition, combining macronutrients in a way that fuels your body efficiently and keeps you feeling satisfied. You'll learn about the importance of portion control and mindful eating, techniques that allow you to enjoy your favorite foods while still making progress towards your goals. We'll also delve into the crucial balance between exercise and rest, showing you how to incorporate physical activity into your routine without burning out or risking injury.

Another central theme is the power of habit formation. Weight loss isn't just about what you eat or how much you exercise; it's about rewiring your brain to make healthier choices automatically. Throughout the 30-day challenge, you'll learn how to build and reinforce positive habits that support your weight loss journey. From meal planning and prep strategies to establishing consistent sleep patterns, you'll develop a toolkit of habits that will serve you long after the challenge is over.

Mindset is another critical component of successful weight loss, and it's a theme that runs throughout this book. We'll address the mental barriers that often hold people back from achieving their weight loss goals, such as negative self-talk, fear of failure, and unrealistic expectations. You'll learn powerful techniques for overcoming these obstacles, cultivating a growth mindset, and staying motivated even when progress seems slow.

Perhaps most importantly, this book emphasizes the importance of sustainability. Too often, weight loss programs focus solely on short-term results, leading to a cycle of yo-yo dieting and frustration. "The Easy Weight Loss Challenge" takes a different approach. While the 30-day program provides a structured starting point, the ultimate goal is to equip you with the knowledge and skills to maintain a healthy lifestyle for years to come. You'll learn how to adapt the principles of the challenge to fit your unique circumstances and preferences, ensuring that your weight loss journey doesn't end after 30 days but evolves into a lifelong commitment to health and wellness.

Who is this book for? In short, it's for anyone who's ready to make a lasting change in their health and body composition. Whether you have 10 pounds to lose or 100, whether you're a fitness novice or someone who's tried every diet under the sun, this book has something to offer you. It's particularly well-suited for busy individuals who need a straightforward, no-nonsense approach to weight loss that fits into their hectic lives. If you're tired of conflicting nutrition advice, complicated workout plans, or programs that require you to buy expensive equipment or supplements, you'll appreciate the simplicity and accessibility of this 30-day challenge.

By the time you finish this book and complete the 30-day challenge, you'll have gained a wealth of knowledge and practical skills. You'll understand the science behind weight loss, including how different foods affect your body and how to leverage exercise for maximum fat-burning potential. You'll have a repertoire of healthy recipes and meal ideas that are not only nutritious but delicious and satisfying. You'll know how to design effective workouts that can be done anywhere, with little to no equipment. Perhaps most importantly, you'll have developed a new relationship with food and your body, one based on self-care and respect rather than deprivation and punishment.

But the benefits extend far beyond just weight loss. As you progress through the challenge, you'll likely notice improvements in your energy levels, sleep quality, and overall mood. Many participants report feeling more confident, both in their appearance and in their ability to tackle other life challenges. You may find that your success in weight loss spills over into other areas of your life, inspiring you to set and achieve new goals in your career, relationships, or personal growth.

One of the unique aspects of "The Easy Weight Loss Challenge" is its emphasis on social support and community. In Chapter 8, we explore how to build a support network that will cheer you on and keep you accountable throughout your weight loss journey. You'll learn strategies for navigating social situations that can often derail weight loss efforts, such as dining out or attending parties. We'll also discuss how to leverage social media and technology to connect with like-minded individuals and access additional resources and motivation.

As you progress through the book, you'll find that each chapter builds upon the last, creating a comprehensive framework for sustainable weight loss. We start with the basics, helping you set realistic goals and prepare mentally and physically for the challenge ahead. From there, we dive into the nitty-gritty of nutrition, exploring macronutrients, calorie counting, and meal planning. You'll learn how to make smart food choices that nourish your body and support your weight loss goals without feeling deprived.

Exercise is, of course, a crucial component of any weight loss program, and we dedicate an entire chapter to helping you find enjoyable ways to move your body. Whether you prefer high-intensity workouts or gentle yoga, we'll show you how to create a fitness routine that fits your lifestyle and preferences. We'll also address often-overlooked factors in weight loss, such as sleep and stress management, providing practical strategies for optimizing these areas of your life.

Throughout the 30-day challenge, we emphasize the importance of tracking your progress and celebrating your successes, no matter how small. You'll learn different methods for measuring your progress beyond just the number on the scale, helping you stay motivated even when weight loss slows down. We also address the common challenge of weight loss plateaus, providing strategies to push through these frustrating periods and continue making progress.

As the 30 days come to a close, we don't leave you hanging. The final chapters of the book focus on maintaining your momentum and transitioning to a long-term healthy lifestyle. You'll learn how to set new goals, handle setbacks, and continue challenging yourself to grow and improve. We also discuss how to inspire others with your success, potentially creating a ripple effect of health and wellness in your community.

By the time you reach the end of this book, you'll have all the tools you need to not just lose weight, but to transform your entire approach to health and wellness. You'll understand that weight loss is not about punishing yourself or adhering to strict rules, but about making informed choices that support your overall well-being. You'll have developed a toolbox of strategies to handle any obstacle that comes your way, from stress-induced cravings to busy schedules that threaten to derail your healthy habits.

Perhaps most importantly, you'll have developed a new sense of confidence and self-efficacy. The 30-day challenge is designed not just to help you lose weight, but to prove to yourself that you're capable of setting a goal and seeing it through. This newfound belief in yourself can be transformative, spilling over into other areas of your life and inspiring you to tackle challenges you may have previously thought impossible.

As you embark on this 30-day journey, remember that every step forward, no matter how small, is progress. There may be days when you struggle or feel like giving up, but know that these challenges are part of the process. Each obstacle you overcome makes you stronger and more resilient. And you're not alone on this journey. Throughout the book, you'll find stories and testimonials from individuals who have successfully completed the challenge, offering inspiration and proof that lasting change is possible.

So, are you ready to take the first step towards a healthier, happier you? Are you prepared to challenge yourself, to push beyond your comfort zone, and to discover what you're truly capable of? If so, turn the page and let's begin this transformative 30-day journey together. Your future self – stronger, healthier, and more confident – is waiting. Let's make the next 30 days the beginning of your new life. Welcome to "The Easy Weight Loss Challenge: 30 Days to a New You." Your transformation starts now.

Chapter 1: Getting Started: Your 30-Day Journey Begins

As we embark on this transformative 30-day weight loss challenge, it's essential to lay a solid foundation for success. This chapter will guide you through the crucial first steps of your journey, helping you understand the concept of a 30-day challenge, set realistic goals, prepare both mentally and physically, and create an environment conducive to achieving your weight loss objectives.

Understanding the 30-day challenge concept is paramount to your success. This approach is rooted in the idea that it takes approximately 21 to 30 days to form a new habit or break an old one. By committing to a focused period of 30 days, you're giving yourself the opportunity to establish new, healthier patterns that can lead to sustainable weight loss. The beauty of a 30-day challenge lies in its defined timeframe, which makes it feel more manageable and less daunting than an open-ended commitment to lose weight.

During these 30 days, you'll be introducing gradual changes to your diet, exercise routine, and lifestyle habits. This approach allows for a more sustainable transformation, as opposed to drastic measures that are often difficult to maintain in the long term. Remember, the goal isn't just to lose weight quickly, but to develop habits that will support your health and well-being for years to come.

One of the key advantages of a 30-day challenge is the momentum it creates. As you progress through the days, you'll likely start to see and feel changes in your body and energy levels. These early wins can be incredibly motivating, propelling you forward and reinforcing your commitment to the process. Moreover, the structured nature of a 30-day program provides a clear roadmap, reducing the overwhelm that often accompanies weight loss attempts.

However, it's crucial to approach this challenge with the right mindset. While 30 days can lead to significant changes, it's not a magic solution. It's the beginning of a journey towards a healthier lifestyle, and the habits you form during this period will serve as the foundation for long-term success.

Setting realistic goals and expectations is a critical step in your 30-day weight loss journey. It's natural to feel excited and ambitious at the start of a new challenge, but it's important to temper that enthusiasm with a dose of realism. Unrealistic expectations can lead to disappointment and demotivation, potentially derailing your efforts before you've had a chance to see real results.

When setting your weight loss goal for the 30-day period, consider the widely accepted healthy rate of weight loss, which is about 1 to 2 pounds per week. This translates to a potential loss of 4 to 8 pounds over the course of the challenge. While this might seem modest compared to the dramatic results promised by fad diets, it's important to remember that slow, steady weight loss is more likely to be sustainable in the long run.

However, weight shouldn't be your only measure of success. Consider setting non-scale goals as well. These might include increasing your daily step count, being able to jog for 10 minutes without stopping, or fitting more comfortably into your clothes. These types of goals can provide motivation and a sense of achievement even when the number on the scale isn't moving as quickly as you'd like.

It's also crucial to set process goals alongside your outcome goals. Process goals focus on the behaviors that will lead to weight loss, rather than the weight loss itself. Examples might include "I will prepare healthy meals at home five nights a week" or "I will exercise for 30 minutes, four times a week." These goals give you more control over your success and help establish the habits that will support long-term weight management.

As you set your goals, be sure to write them down. Research has shown that the act of writing down goals increases the likelihood of achieving them. Be specific about what you want to achieve and by when. Instead of a vague goal like "lose weight," try something like "lose 6 pounds in 30 days by following the meal plan and exercising 4 times a week."

Remember, the purpose of this 30-day challenge is not just to lose weight, but to kickstart a healthier lifestyle. Your ultimate goal should be to feel better, have more energy, and develop habits that you can maintain beyond the 30 days. Keep this bigger picture in mind as you set your expectations for the challenge.

Preparing mentally and physically for the journey ahead is a crucial step that many people overlook when starting a weight loss program. The mental aspect of weight loss is just as important, if not more so, than the physical component. Your mindset can make the difference between giving up when faced with obstacles and pushing through to achieve your goals.

Start by examining your motivation for wanting to lose weight. Is it to improve your health? To feel more confident? To have more energy to play with your kids? Understanding your "why" can provide powerful motivation when the going gets tough. Write down your reasons and keep them somewhere visible as a daily reminder of what you're working towards.

It's also important to address any negative self-talk or limiting beliefs you might have about your ability to lose weight. Many people have a history of failed diets or weight loss attempts, which can lead to a defeatist attitude. Challenge these thoughts by reminding yourself that this time is different. You're not just going on another diet; you're making a commitment to change your lifestyle for the better.

Visualization can be a powerful tool in preparing mentally for your weight loss journey. Spend some time each day visualizing yourself successfully completing the 30-day challenge. Imagine how you'll look and feel at the end of the 30 days, and the sense of accomplishment you'll experience. This practice can help build confidence and reinforce your commitment to the process.

Physical preparation is equally important. Before diving into a new exercise routine, it's wise to consult with your healthcare provider, especially if you have any pre-existing health conditions or if it's been a while since you've engaged in regular physical activity. They can provide guidance on any precautions you should take and might even offer suggestions tailored to your specific health needs.

Start preparing your body by gradually increasing your daily activity level. This could be as simple as taking a short walk each day or doing some gentle stretching. The goal is to start building the habit of regular movement and to prepare your body for the increased activity level you'll be undertaking during the challenge.

Hydration is another key aspect of physical preparation. Many people are chronically dehydrated, which can impact energy levels and even mimic hunger. In the days leading up to the challenge, focus on increasing your water intake. A good rule of thumb is to aim for eight 8-ounce glasses of water per day, but individual needs may vary based on factors like activity level and climate.

Lastly, consider doing a kitchen clean-out. Remove or reduce tempting, unhealthy foods from your environment. While you don't need to completely eliminate all treats, having them easily accessible can make it harder to stick to your goals, especially in the early days of the challenge when you're still building new habits.

Creating a supportive environment for success is a critical yet often overlooked aspect of any weight loss journey. Your environment plays a significant role in shaping your behaviors and can either support or hinder your efforts to lose weight. By intentionally structuring your surroundings to align with your goals, you can set yourself up for success right from the start of your 30-day challenge.

Begin by assessing your home environment, particularly your kitchen. As mentioned earlier, a kitchen clean-out can be beneficial. However, it's not just about removing unhealthy foods; it's also about stocking up on nutritious options. Fill your fridge with fresh fruits and vegetables, lean proteins, and whole grains. Having healthy foods readily available makes it easier to make good choices, even when you're tired or pressed for time.

Consider reorganizing your kitchen to make healthy choices more convenient. Place a fruit bowl in a prominent location for easy snacking. Store your healthiest foods at eye level in the fridge and pantry, making them the first things you see when you open the door. Conversely, if you choose to keep some less healthy items in the house, store them out of sight, perhaps on a high shelf or in a less accessible location.

Your workspace, whether at home or in an office, is another important environment to consider. If you tend to snack while working, stock your desk drawer with healthy options like nuts or dried fruit. Keep a water bottle within reach to encourage regular hydration. If you have control over your work schedule, consider blocking out time for short walks or stretching sessions throughout the day.

Technology can also play a role in creating a supportive environment. Consider downloading apps that can help you track your food intake, monitor your exercise, or provide motivation and support. Set reminders on your phone for meal prep, exercise sessions, or even to take a moment for mindful breathing or stress relief.

Social media can be a double-edged sword when it comes to weight loss. On one hand, it can provide inspiration and support. On the other, it can expose you to unrealistic body images or tempting food photos. Consider curating your social media feeds to follow accounts that align with your health goals and unfollowing or muting those that don't.

Your social environment is equally important. Inform your friends and family about your 30-day challenge and ask for their support. This could mean asking them to respect your food choices, inviting them to join you for workouts, or simply requesting their encouragement. If possible, find a buddy who wants to take on the challenge with you. Having someone to share the journey with can provide accountability and make the process more enjoyable.

Creating a supportive sleep environment is also crucial, given the important role that sleep plays in weight management. Make your bedroom a sanctuary for rest. Invest in comfortable bedding, use blackout curtains if needed, and consider removing electronic devices from the bedroom to reduce sleep disruptions.

Remember, creating a supportive environment is an ongoing process. As you progress through your 30-day challenge, you may identify new ways to optimize your surroundings to better support your goals. Be open to making adjustments as you learn what works best for you.

As we conclude this chapter on getting started with your 30-day weight loss journey, it's important to remember that the steps we've discussed – understanding the challenge concept, setting realistic goals, preparing mentally and physically, and creating a supportive environment – are foundational to your success. They set the stage for the specific strategies and tactics we'll explore in the coming chapters.

The journey you're about to embark on is about more than just losing weight. It's about taking control of your health, developing sustainable habits, and improving your overall quality of life. As you move forward, keep in mind that this 30-day challenge is just the beginning. The habits and knowledge you gain during this time will serve as building blocks for a healthier lifestyle that extends far beyond these 30 days.

In the next chapter, we'll delve into the fundamentals of nutrition and how to fuel your body effectively for weight loss. You'll learn about macronutrients, calorie counting, the importance of hydration, and strategies for meal planning and preparation. These nutritional basics will form a crucial part of your weight loss toolkit, complementing the foundational work you've done in this first chapter. Remember, each step you take brings you closer to your goals, and with the right knowledge and preparation, you're well on your way to becoming a healthier, more energetic version of yourself.

Chapter 2: Nutrition Basics: Fueling Your Body for Weight Loss

As we embark on the next phase of our 30-day weight loss journey, it's crucial to understand that nutrition plays a pivotal role in achieving our goals. The food we consume is not merely fuel for our bodies; it's the foundation upon which we build our health and well-being. In this chapter, we'll delve into the fundamentals of nutrition that will empower you to make informed choices and set you on the path to successful weight loss.

Understanding macronutrients and their role in weight loss

Macronutrients are the building blocks of our diet, consisting of carbohydrates, proteins, and fats. Each of these plays a unique and essential role in our body's functions and, when balanced correctly, can significantly impact our weight loss efforts.

Carbohydrates are often misunderstood in the context of weight loss. While some diets demonize carbs, they are, in fact, our body's primary source of energy. Complex carbohydrates, found in whole grains, vegetables, and legumes, provide sustained energy and are rich in fiber, which aids in digestion and promotes feelings of fullness. On the other hand, simple carbohydrates, typically found in processed foods and sugary drinks, can lead to rapid spikes in blood sugar and contribute to weight gain when consumed in excess.

Proteins are crucial for weight loss as they help build and repair tissues, including muscle. When we're in a calorie deficit for weight loss, adequate protein intake ensures that we lose fat rather than muscle mass. Protein also has a high thermic effect, meaning our bodies burn more calories digesting protein compared to carbs or fats. Good sources of protein include lean meats, fish, eggs, dairy, and plant-based options like legumes and tofu.

Fats, contrary to popular belief, are not the enemy of weight loss. Healthy fats are essential for hormone production, nutrient absorption, and brain function. They also contribute to satiety, helping you feel full and satisfied after meals. Sources of healthy fats include avocados, nuts, seeds, olive oil, and fatty fish. However, it's important to consume fats in moderation due to their high calorie content.

Understanding the role of each macronutrient allows us to create balanced meals that support our weight loss goals while ensuring our bodies receive the nutrients they need to function optimally. As Dr. David Ludwig, professor of nutrition at Harvard School of Public Health, states, "The quality of the calories you consume is just as important as the quantity when it comes to weight management and overall health."

Simple calorie counting techniques

While the quality of our food is paramount, the quantity still matters when it comes to weight loss. At its core, weight loss occurs when we consume fewer calories than we burn. However, calorie counting doesn't have to be a complex or time-consuming process.

One simple technique is the hand portion method. This approach uses your hand as a measuring tool, making it easy to estimate portion sizes without the need for scales or measuring cups. For example, a serving of protein should be about the size and thickness of your palm, a serving of carbohydrates can fit in your cupped hand, and a serving of vegetables is roughly the size of your fist. This method allows for flexibility and can be used even when dining out or in social situations.

Another effective technique is the plate method. This involves visually dividing your plate into sections: half of your plate should be filled with non-starchy vegetables, a quarter with lean protein, and the remaining quarter with complex carbohydrates. This simple visual guide ensures a balanced meal without the need for precise measurements.

For those who prefer a more structured approach, numerous smartphone apps can help track calorie intake. These apps often have extensive food databases, making it easy to log meals and snacks. However, it's important to use these tools as guides rather than strict rules. Nutritionist Rhiannon Lambert advises, "While calorie counting can be a useful tool for some, it's essential to focus on the nutritional value of foods rather than just their calorie content. A balanced, varied diet is key to sustainable weight loss."

Importance of hydration in weight loss

Water is often overlooked in weight loss discussions, but its importance cannot be overstated. Proper hydration is crucial for numerous bodily functions, including metabolism and the transportation of nutrients. Moreover, staying well-hydrated can significantly aid in weight loss efforts.

Drinking water before meals can help reduce calorie intake by promoting feelings of fullness. A study published in the journal Obesity found that adults who drank water before meals lost 44% more weight over a 12-week period compared to those who didn't. Water can also boost metabolism temporarily. Research has shown that drinking 500ml of water increases resting metabolism by 24-30% for up to an hour.

Often, thirst can be mistaken for hunger, leading to unnecessary snacking. By staying hydrated throughout the day, we can better distinguish between true hunger and thirst, potentially reducing overall calorie intake. Aim to drink at least 8 glasses (64 ounces) of water per day, and more if you're physically active or in hot weather.

It's not just about quantity, but also about timing. Starting your day with a glass of water can help kickstart your metabolism and rehydrate your body after hours of sleep. Drinking water between meals, rather than with meals, can aid digestion and nutrient absorption.

While water should be your primary source of hydration, other beverages like herbal teas and infused waters can contribute to your daily fluid intake while adding variety. However, be cautious with drinks that contain calories, such as fruit juices and smoothies, as these can quickly add up and hinder weight loss efforts if not accounted for in your overall calorie intake.

Meal planning and prep strategies for busy lifestyles

One of the biggest challenges in maintaining a healthy diet for weight loss is navigating busy schedules and the temptation of convenient, often unhealthy, food options. Meal planning and preparation can be powerful tools in overcoming these obstacles, setting you up for success throughout your weight loss journey.

Meal planning involves deciding your meals in advance, typically for a week at a time. This practice not only saves time and reduces stress during the week but also helps ensure you have balanced, nutritious meals aligned with your weight loss goals. Start by setting aside time each week, perhaps on a Sunday evening, to plan your meals for the upcoming week. Consider your schedule, including any social engagements or late workdays, and plan accordingly.

When meal planning, aim for variety to ensure you're getting a wide range of nutrients and to prevent boredom. Include a mix of proteins, complex carbohydrates, and plenty of vegetables in your meals. Don't forget to plan for snacks as well, as these can often be the downfall of an otherwise healthy eating plan.

Once you have your meal plan, create a comprehensive shopping list. This not only saves time at the grocery store but also helps prevent impulse purchases of unhealthy foods. Stick to the perimeter of the store where fresh, whole foods are typically located, and be cautious when venturing into the inner aisles where processed foods often reside.

Meal preparation, or "meal prep," takes planning a step further by preparing some or all of your meals in advance. This could involve cooking large batches of food to portion out for the week, preparing ingredients for quick assembly later, or even fully preparing meals to reheat throughout the week.

A common meal prep strategy is to dedicate a few hours on the weekend to cook several meals for the week ahead. For example, you might roast a large batch of vegetables, grill several chicken breasts, and cook a pot of quinoa. These components can then be mixed and matched throughout the week for varied meals. Store these prepped foods in clear containers in your refrigerator for easy access.

For busy mornings, overnight oats or chia seed puddings can be prepared in advance and grabbed on the go. Salad jars are another great option for prepared lunches - layer dressing at the bottom, followed by hardy vegetables, proteins, and finally leafy greens on top to keep everything fresh.

Remember, meal prep doesn't have to mean eating the same thing every day. You can prepare versatile ingredients that can be used in different ways throughout the week. For instance, grilled chicken can be used in salads, wraps, or stirfries.

Registered dietitian Toby Amidor emphasizes the importance of meal prep, stating, "Meal prepping is a critical tool for weight loss success. It puts you in control of your food choices and portions, reducing the likelihood of impulsive, often less healthy food decisions when you're pressed for time or energy."

While meal planning and prep require some upfront time and effort, they can save significant time and stress during the week. More importantly, they provide a structured approach to nutrition that supports your weight loss goals, even amidst a hectic lifestyle.

As we conclude this chapter on nutrition basics, it's important to remember that these principles form the foundation of your weight loss journey. Understanding macronutrients, implementing simple calorie counting techniques, prioritizing hydration, and mastering meal planning and prep are key skills that will serve you well beyond the 30-day challenge.

In the next chapter, we'll build upon these nutritional basics and explore smart eating habits that can lead to significant results. We'll delve into portion control techniques, mindful eating practices, and strategies for dealing with cravings and emotional eating. These practical skills will further empower you to make sustainable changes to your eating habits, bringing you closer to your weight loss goals.

Remember, the journey to weight loss and better health is not about perfection, but progress. As you implement these nutrition basics, be patient with yourself and celebrate the small victories along the way. Each healthy choice you make is a step towards the new you that you're working to become.

Chapter 3: Smart Eating Habits: Small Changes, Big Results

As we transition from the foundational aspects of nutrition covered in the previous chapter, it's time to delve into the practical application of smart eating habits. These habits, seemingly small and insignificant on their own, can accumulate to create substantial changes in your weight loss journey. The beauty of these strategies lies in their simplicity and ease of implementation, making them perfect for our 30-day challenge.

Portion control is perhaps one of the most crucial yet often overlooked aspects of weight management. In today's supersized world, our perception of what constitutes a normal portion has become severely distorted. Restaurants serve plates piled high with food, and packaged snacks often contain multiple servings in a single container. This abundance of food has led to a phenomenon known as "portion distortion," where we consistently overeat without even realizing it.

To combat this, it's essential to educate ourselves on what appropriate portion sizes look like. A simple rule of thumb is to use your hand as a guide. Your palm can represent a serving of protein, your fist a serving of vegetables, your cupped hand a serving of carbohydrates, and your thumb a serving of fats. This method is particularly useful when eating out or in situations where measuring tools aren't readily available.

Another effective technique is to use smaller plates and bowls. This simple change can trick your brain into feeling satisfied with less food. Studies have shown that people tend to eat 92% of what they serve themselves, regardless of the plate size. By using smaller dinnerware, you naturally serve yourself less, leading to reduced calorie intake without feeling deprived.

It's also crucial to be mindful of high-calorie condiments and dressings. These can add significant calories to an otherwise healthy meal. For instance, a tablespoon of mayonnaise contains around 90 calories, while the same amount of olive oil has 120 calories. Instead of eliminating these entirely, try using them sparingly or opting for lower-calorie alternatives like mustard, vinegar, or lemon juice.

Mindful eating is another powerful tool in your weight loss arsenal. In our fast-paced society, we often eat on the go, in front of screens, or while multitasking. This distracted eating can lead to overconsumption and a disconnection from our body's hunger and fullness cues. Mindful eating encourages us to slow down, savor our food, and pay attention to our body's signals.

To practice mindful eating, start by removing distractions during mealtimes. Turn off the TV, put away your phone, and focus solely on your meal. Take the time to appreciate the colors, smells, and textures of your food before you begin eating. As you eat, chew slowly and thoroughly, paying attention to the flavors and sensations in your mouth.

Dr. Jan Chozen Bays, author of "Mindful Eating: A Guide to Rediscovering a Healthy and Joyful Relationship with Food," emphasizes the importance of this practice: "Mindful eating replaces automatic eating with conscious eating. It's about being aware of what you're eating, why you're eating, and how it affects your body and mind."

Another aspect of mindful eating is learning to recognize true hunger versus emotional or habitual eating. Before reaching for food, pause and ask yourself if you're genuinely hungry or if you're eating for other reasons such as boredom, stress, or habit. If you're not physically hungry, try engaging in a different activity or addressing the underlying emotion directly.

Healthy snacking is an essential component of any successful weight loss plan. Contrary to popular belief, snacking can actually aid in weight loss when done correctly. Smart snacking can help maintain stable blood sugar levels, prevent overeating at meals, and provide necessary nutrients throughout the day.

The key to healthy snacking is preparation and planning. Keep a variety of nutritious, portion-controlled snacks readily available. This could include fresh fruits, cut vegetables with hummus, a small handful of nuts, or Greek yogurt with berries. By having these options on hand, you're less likely to reach for unhealthy alternatives when hunger strikes.

When choosing snacks, aim for a combination of protein and fiber. This pairing helps keep you feeling full and satisfied. For example, an apple with a tablespoon of almond butter, or carrot sticks with a quarter cup of guacamole. These combinations provide a balance of nutrients and help curb hunger until your next meal.

It's also important to be mindful of liquid calories when snacking. Many beverages, including sodas, fruit juices, and fancy coffee drinks, can contain a significant amount of hidden calories and sugar. Opt for water, unsweetened tea, or black coffee instead. If you need some flavor, try infusing water with fresh fruits or herbs for a refreshing, calorie-free drink.

Dealing with cravings and emotional eating is often one of the most challenging aspects of weight loss. It's crucial to understand that cravings are normal and don't necessarily indicate a lack of willpower. Often, cravings are triggered by emotions, habits, or environmental cues rather than genuine hunger.

When faced with a craving, the first step is to pause and identify the trigger. Are you stressed, bored, or tired? Once you've identified the underlying cause, you can address it directly. If you're stressed, try a quick relaxation technique like deep breathing or a short walk. If you're bored, engage in a hobby or call a friend. By addressing the root cause, you may find that the craving passes.

If the craving persists, try the "delay and distract" technique. Tell yourself you'll wait 15 minutes before indulging. During this time, engage in a distracting activity. Often, you'll find that the craving has passed by the end of the waiting period. If you still want the food after the delay, allow yourself to have a small portion, savoring it mindfully.

It's also helpful to examine your food environment. Remove tempting, unhealthy foods from your home and replace them with nutritious alternatives. This doesn't mean you can never enjoy treats, but by making them less accessible, you reduce the likelihood of impulsive eating.

Emotional eating is a common challenge for many people trying to lose weight. It involves using food to cope with emotions rather than to satisfy physical hunger. To combat emotional eating, it's essential to develop alternative coping mechanisms. This could include journaling, practicing meditation, engaging in physical activity, or talking to a supportive friend or therapist.

Dr. Susan Albers, a psychologist and expert on mindful eating, suggests: "Instead of trying to fight or ignore your emotions, work on accepting them. Emotional acceptance doesn't mean you like the emotion, but that you acknowledge it without judgment. This can help reduce the urge to eat in response to feelings."

As we conclude this chapter on smart eating habits, it's important to remember that these changes don't need to be drastic or happen all at once. Small, consistent changes can lead to significant results over time. Be patient with yourself as you implement these new habits, and remember that perfection is not the goal. The key is progress and consistency.

As we move forward in our 30-day challenge, we'll build upon these smart eating habits by exploring the role of exercise in weight loss. Physical activity not only burns calories but also boosts metabolism, improves mood, and enhances overall health. In the next chapter, we'll discover how to incorporate enjoyable and effective exercise into your daily routine, even if you're new to working out or have a busy schedule. Remember, every step you take, no matter how small, brings you closer to your weight loss goals and a healthier lifestyle.

Chapter 4: Exercise Essentials: Moving Your Way to a Slimmer You

As we transition from our discussion on smart eating habits, it's time to delve into another crucial aspect of your weight loss journey: exercise. While nutrition plays a significant role in shedding those extra pounds, incorporating regular physical activity into your routine can accelerate your progress and provide numerous additional health benefits.

Benefits of regular exercise for weight loss

Exercise is not just about burning calories; it's a transformative tool that can reshape your body and mind. When you engage in physical activity, your body undergoes a series of positive changes that contribute to weight loss and overall well-being. One of the primary benefits of exercise is its ability to boost your metabolism. As you move your body, you increase your muscle mass, which in turn raises your basal metabolic rate. This means you'll burn more calories even when you're at rest.

Moreover, exercise helps to preserve lean muscle mass during weight loss. When you're in a calorie deficit, your body may break down muscle tissue for energy. However, by incorporating strength training into your routine, you can signal to your body to retain muscle while primarily burning fat for fuel. This is crucial for maintaining a healthy metabolism and achieving a toned, sculpted appearance.

Regular physical activity also improves insulin sensitivity, which is essential for managing blood sugar levels and preventing type 2 diabetes. As your body becomes more efficient at utilizing insulin, it's less likely to store excess glucose as fat, further supporting your weight loss efforts. Additionally, exercise has been shown to reduce visceral fat, the dangerous fat that accumulates around your organs and is associated with numerous health risks.

Beyond the physical benefits, exercise has a profound impact on your mental health. It triggers the release of endorphins, often referred to as "feel-good" hormones, which can elevate your mood and reduce stress. This psychological boost can be particularly valuable during your weight loss journey, helping you stay motivated and resilient in the face of challenges.

Exercise also improves sleep quality, which, as we'll discuss in a later chapter, plays a crucial role in weight management. Regular physical activity can help you fall asleep faster and enjoy deeper, more restorative sleep. This, in turn, can regulate hormones that influence appetite and metabolism, creating a positive cycle that supports your weight loss goals.

It's important to note that the benefits of exercise extend far beyond weight loss. Regular physical activity strengthens your heart, improves lung function, and enhances overall cardiovascular health. It can lower blood pressure, reduce the risk of certain cancers, and even boost cognitive function. By incorporating exercise into your 30-day challenge, you're not just working towards a slimmer you; you're investing in your long-term health and vitality.

Simple at-home workout routines

Now that we understand the myriad benefits of exercise, let's explore some simple at-home workout routines that you can incorporate into your daily life. The beauty of these routines is that they require minimal equipment and can be adapted to suit various fitness levels.

Begin with a basic bodyweight circuit that targets all major muscle groups. Start with 10-15 squats, which work your lower body and core. Follow this with 10-15 push-ups (you can do these on your knees if needed) to engage your chest, shoulders, and arms. Next, perform 10-15 lunges on each leg to further challenge your lower body. Complete the circuit with 30 seconds of high knees or jogging in place for a cardiovascular boost. Repeat this circuit 3-4 times, resting for 30-60 seconds between each round.

As you progress, you can increase the number of repetitions or add more challenging variations. For instance, you might try jump squats instead of regular squats, or diamond push-ups to further target your triceps. The key is to continually challenge yourself while maintaining proper form to prevent injury.

Another effective at-home workout is the Tabata protocol, a form of high-intensity interval training (HIIT). Choose an exercise, such as mountain climbers, and perform it at maximum effort for 20 seconds, followed by 10 seconds of rest. Repeat this 8 times for a total of 4 minutes. This intense workout can be incredibly effective for burning calories and improving cardiovascular fitness in a short amount of time.

For those who prefer a more gentle approach, consider incorporating yoga into your routine. A sun salutation sequence, performed for 10-15 minutes each morning, can help improve flexibility, build strength, and center your mind for the day ahead. As you become more comfortable with the poses, you can explore more challenging sequences or longer sessions.

Remember, consistency is key when it comes to at-home workouts. It's better to do a 15-minute workout every day than to attempt a grueling 2-hour session once a week. Set aside a specific time each day for your workout, and treat it as a non-negotiable appointment with yourself. This will help you establish a routine and make exercise a habit rather than a chore.

Incorporating cardio and strength training

While bodyweight exercises provide an excellent foundation for your fitness routine, it's important to incorporate both cardio and strength training for optimal weight loss results. Cardiovascular exercise, or cardio, is crucial for burning calories, improving heart health, and boosting your overall endurance. Strength training, on the other hand, helps build lean muscle mass, which increases your metabolism and gives your body a more toned appearance.

For cardio, consider activities that elevate your heart rate and can be sustained for at least 20-30 minutes. If you have access to outdoor spaces, brisk walking, jogging, or cycling are excellent options. Start with 20-30 minutes of moderate-intensity cardio, 3-4 times a week. As your fitness improves, you can increase the duration or intensity of your sessions.

If you prefer indoor cardio, there are numerous options available. Jumping rope is a highly effective cardio workout that also improves coordination and agility. Start with short intervals, such as 30 seconds of jumping followed by 30 seconds of rest, and gradually increase your jumping time as you build endurance. Dancing is another fun and effective form of cardio that can be done at home. Put on your favorite upbeat music and dance for 20-30 minutes, focusing on continuous movement and using your whole body.

For strength training, you don't need a fully equipped gym to see results. Resistance bands are an affordable and versatile tool that can provide effective strength workouts at home. Use them to add resistance to exercises like squats, bicep curls, and rows. If you don't have resistance bands, household items can serve as makeshift weights. Filled water bottles, cans of food, or even books can be used for exercises like overhead presses or lateral raises.

To create a balanced routine, aim to include both cardio and strength training in your weekly schedule. For example, you might do cardio on Monday, Wednesday, and Friday, and strength training on Tuesday and Thursday. Remember to allow for rest days to give your body time to recover and prevent burnout.

As you progress in your fitness journey, consider incorporating more advanced techniques like supersets or circuit training. These methods involve performing exercises back-to-back with minimal rest, which can help boost calorie burn and improve overall fitness. However, it's crucial to build a solid foundation of proper form and technique before attempting more intense workouts.

Finding enjoyable physical activities to stay motivated

While structured workouts are important, the key to long-term success is finding physical activities that you genuinely enjoy. When exercise feels like a chore, it's easy to lose motivation and fall off track. By discovering activities that bring you joy, you're more likely to stick with them and make physical activity a permanent part of your lifestyle.

Consider exploring different types of movement to find what resonates with you. If you enjoy music and rhythmic movement, try dance-based workouts like Zumba or hip-hop fitness classes. Many of these are available online and can be done in the comfort of your own home. If you prefer a more meditative approach, practices like tai chi or qigong combine gentle movements with mindfulness, providing both physical and mental benefits.

For those who thrive on competition or social interaction, consider joining online fitness challenges or virtual workout groups. Many fitness apps and social media platforms offer communities where you can connect with like-minded individuals, share progress, and participate in friendly competitions. This sense of community can provide accountability and motivation, making your fitness journey more enjoyable and sustainable.

Nature lovers might find joy in outdoor activities like hiking, kayaking, or rock climbing. While these may not be daily exercises, incorporating them into your weekends or free time can provide a refreshing change of pace and help you stay active in a way that doesn't feel like traditional exercise.

Don't be afraid to think outside the box when it comes to physical activity. Activities like gardening, playing with your children or pets, or even active video games can contribute to your daily movement goals. The key is to find ways to make movement a natural and enjoyable part of your daily life.

Remember that your preferences may change over time, and that's okay. Be open to trying new activities and revisiting ones you may have dismissed in the past. Your body and mindset will evolve throughout your weight loss journey, and activities that once seemed challenging or unenjoyable might become your new favorites.

As we conclude this chapter on exercise essentials, it's important to emphasize that movement is a celebration of what your body can do, not a punishment for what you ate. Approach exercise with a positive mindset, focusing on how it makes you feel rather than solely on its calorie-burning potential. As you progress through your 30-day challenge, you'll likely find that the benefits of regular physical activity extend far beyond weight loss, enhancing your overall quality of life.

In the next chapter, we'll explore the often-overlooked factors of sleep and stress management in your weight loss journey. These elements play a crucial role in your overall health and can significantly impact your ability to achieve and maintain your weight loss goals. By addressing these areas, you'll be equipped with a comprehensive approach to transforming your body and lifestyle.

Chapter 5: Sleep and Stress: The Hidden Factors in Weight Loss

As we transition from our discussion on exercise essentials, it's crucial to recognize that weight loss isn't solely about diet and physical activity. Two often overlooked yet significant factors in the weight loss equation are sleep and stress. These elements play a pivotal role in our body's ability to shed excess pounds and maintain a healthy weight. In this chapter, we'll explore the intricate relationship between sleep, stress, and weight loss, and provide practical strategies to optimize these areas for your weight loss journey.

Understanding the impact of sleep on weight loss

Sleep is not merely a period of rest for our bodies; it's an active time of restoration, repair, and regulation of various bodily functions, including those related to weight management. When we don't get enough quality sleep, our body's intricate hormonal balance is disrupted, leading to a cascade of effects that can sabotage our weight loss efforts.

One of the primary ways lack of sleep impacts weight is through its effect on hunger hormones. Ghrelin, often called the "hunger hormone," increases when we're sleep-deprived, while leptin, the hormone that signals fullness, decreases. This hormonal imbalance can lead to increased appetite and cravings, particularly for high-calorie, carbohydrate-rich foods. Dr. Eve Van Cauter, a sleep researcher at the University of Chicago, found that people who slept only four hours a night for two nights had a 24% increase in hunger compared to those who slept ten hours a night.

Moreover, insufficient sleep affects our body's ability to regulate blood sugar levels. A study published in the Annals of Internal Medicine revealed that just four days of sleep deprivation reduced insulin sensitivity by more than 30%. This reduction in insulin sensitivity can lead to increased fat storage and difficulty losing weight.

Sleep deprivation also impacts our decision-making abilities and willpower. When we're tired, we're more likely to make poor food choices, skip workouts, and give in to temptations. This is partly due to the fact that sleep deprivation affects the prefrontal cortex, the part of our brain responsible for self-control and decision-making.

Furthermore, lack of sleep can lead to increased cortisol levels, often referred to as the "stress hormone." Elevated cortisol levels can promote fat storage, particularly around the abdominal area. This visceral fat is not only aesthetically undesirable but also poses significant health risks.

It's clear that prioritizing sleep is not a luxury but a necessity for effective weight loss. Aim for 7-9 hours of quality sleep per night to support your body's natural weight regulation processes. Remember, sleep is not a passive state; it's an active time when your body is working hard to support your weight loss goals.

Stress management techniques for better weight control

Stress, like inadequate sleep, can be a significant roadblock in your weight loss journey. Chronic stress can lead to weight gain and difficulty losing weight through various mechanisms. Understanding these connections and implementing effective stress management techniques can significantly enhance your weight loss efforts.

When we're stressed, our body releases cortisol, which, as mentioned earlier, can promote fat storage, especially around the midsection. Additionally, stress can lead to emotional eating, where food becomes a coping mechanism rather than a source of nourishment. This often results in overconsumption of high-calorie, low-nutrient foods.

Stress can also interfere with our sleep patterns, creating a vicious cycle that further impacts our weight loss efforts. It's essential to break this cycle by implementing stress management techniques. Here are several effective strategies:

Mindfulness meditation is a powerful tool for managing stress. This practice involves focusing on the present moment without judgment. A study published in the Journal of Obesity found that mindfulness-based interventions were effective for weight loss and improving obesity-related eating behaviors. Start with just five minutes a day and gradually increase your practice.

Regular exercise is another excellent stress-buster. Physical activity releases endorphins, the body's natural mood elevators. It also provides a healthy outlet for stress and tension. Remember, exercise doesn't have to be intense to be effective for stress relief. Even a brisk walk or gentle yoga session can significantly reduce stress levels.

Deep breathing exercises can quickly activate your body's relaxation response. The 4-7-8 technique, developed by Dr. Andrew Weil, is particularly effective. Inhale for a count of 4, hold for 7, and exhale for 8. Repeat this cycle four times. This simple practice can be done anywhere, anytime you feel stress levels rising.

Progressive muscle relaxation is another useful technique. This involves tensing and then relaxing different muscle groups in your body, promoting physical and mental relaxation. Start from your toes and work your way up to your head, tensing each muscle group for 5 seconds before releasing.

Engaging in hobbies or activities you enjoy can also be an effective stress management tool. Whether it's reading, gardening, painting, or playing music, these activities can provide a much-needed mental break and reduce stress levels.

Social support is crucial for managing stress. Talking to friends, family, or a therapist can provide emotional relief and new perspectives on stressful situations. Don't hesitate to reach out when you're feeling overwhelmed.

Time management techniques can also help reduce stress by increasing your sense of control over your daily life. Prioritize tasks, break large projects into smaller, manageable steps, and don't be afraid to delegate when possible.

Remember, stress management is a skill that improves with practice. Be patient with yourself as you explore different techniques and find what works best for you. The goal is to create a toolbox of stress management strategies that you can draw from as needed.

Creating a sleep-friendly environment

Now that we understand the crucial role of sleep in weight loss, let's explore how to create an environment that promotes quality sleep. Your bedroom should be a sanctuary dedicated to rest and relaxation. Here are some key elements to consider:

Temperature plays a significant role in sleep quality. The National Sleep Foundation recommends keeping your bedroom between 60-67°F (15-19°C) for optimal sleep. Our body temperature naturally drops as we prepare for sleep, and a cool room can facilitate this process.

Darkness is essential for promoting the production of melatonin, our sleep hormone. Use blackout curtains or an eye mask to block out light.

If you need a night light, opt for red light, which has the least impact on melatonin production.

Noise can significantly disrupt sleep. If you live in a noisy environment, consider using a white noise machine or earplugs to create a quieter sleep environment. Some people find that nature sounds or soft, ambient music can also promote relaxation and sleep.

Your mattress and pillows play a crucial role in sleep quality. Invest in a comfortable, supportive mattress and pillows that align your spine properly. Remember, what works for one person may not work for another, so choose based on your personal comfort preferences.

Keep electronics out of the bedroom. The blue light emitted by phones, tablets, and computers can interfere with melatonin production. Try to avoid screens for at least an hour before bed. If you must use devices, consider using blue light blocking glasses or apps that filter out blue light.

Establish a relaxing bedtime routine. This might include activities like reading a book, taking a warm bath, or practicing gentle stretches. A consistent routine signals to your body that it's time to wind down and prepare for sleep.

Consider the scents in your bedroom. Lavender has been shown to promote relaxation and improve sleep quality. You could use a lavender-scented pillow spray or essential oil diffuser to create a calming atmosphere.

Keep your bedroom clutter-free. A tidy, organized space can promote a sense of calm and reduce stress, making it easier to relax and fall asleep.

By creating a sleep-friendly environment, you're setting the stage for quality rest, which in turn supports your weight loss efforts. Remember, small changes can make a big difference when it comes to improving sleep quality.

Balancing work, life, and weight loss goals

In our fast-paced modern world, finding balance between work, personal life, and health goals can seem like an insurmountable challenge. However, achieving this balance is crucial for sustainable weight loss and overall well-being. Let's explore strategies to help you juggle these different aspects of your life while staying committed to your weight loss journey.

First and foremost, it's essential to recognize that balance doesn't mean giving equal time to all areas of your life every day. Instead, it's about ensuring that over time, you're giving adequate attention to all important aspects of your life. Some days may be work-heavy, while others may allow more time for personal activities and health goals.

Time management is a critical skill in achieving balance. Start by auditing how you currently spend your time. Are there activities that don't align with your priorities or goals? Can you eliminate or reduce time spent on these? Use tools like calendars or time-tracking apps to help you visualize your time allocation.

Prioritization is key. Stephen Covey, author of "The 7 Habits of Highly Effective People," suggests categorizing tasks into four quadrants based on urgency and importance. Focus on tasks that are important but not urgent, as these often relate to long-term goals and personal development, including your health and weight loss objectives.

Learn to set boundaries. This applies to both work and personal life. It's okay to say no to additional work tasks or social engagements if they interfere with your health goals. Remember, taking care of your health is not selfish; it's necessary for long-term productivity and happiness.

Integrate your weight loss goals into your daily routine. For instance, use your lunch break for a quick workout, or have walking meetings instead of sitting in a conference room. Prepare healthy meals in bulk on weekends to save time during busy weekdays. These small integrations can make a big difference without requiring significant time commitments.

Leverage technology to your advantage. Use apps for meal planning, workout tracking, and meditation. These tools can help you stay on track with minimal time investment.

Practice mindfulness throughout your day. This doesn't mean you need to meditate for hours. Even taking a few deep breaths before responding to an email or savoring your food during meals can help reduce stress and keep you connected to your goals.

Remember the importance of sleep in this equation. It might be tempting to cut back on sleep to fit everything in, but this will likely backfire. Adequate sleep is crucial for managing stress, maintaining willpower, and supporting your body's weight loss efforts.

Be flexible and kind to yourself. There will be days when things don't go as planned. Instead of viewing these as failures, see them as learning opportunities. What can you do differently next time? How can you adapt your plan to better fit your life?

Regularly reassess and adjust your approach. What works during one phase of your life may not work in another. Be open to changing your strategies as your life circumstances evolve.

Remember, achieving balance is an ongoing process, not a destination. It requires constant adjustment and fine-tuning. By implementing these strategies and remaining committed to your goals, you can create a sustainable approach to weight loss that fits within the context of your busy life.

As we conclude this chapter on sleep and stress, it's clear that these factors play a crucial role in your weight loss journey. By prioritizing quality sleep, managing stress effectively, creating a sleep-friendly environment, and finding balance in your life, you're setting yourself up for success. These elements work synergistically with proper nutrition and exercise to create a holistic approach to weight loss.

In the next chapter, we'll explore various methods to track your progress on this 30-day challenge. Remember, weight loss is not just about the number on the scale, and we'll discuss how to measure success in multiple ways. This comprehensive approach to tracking progress will help you stay motivated and make informed decisions as you continue on your journey to a healthier you.

Chapter 6: Tracking Progress: Measuring Success Beyond the Scale

As we transition from the discussion on sleep and stress management in the previous chapter, it's important to recognize that weight loss is a multifaceted journey. While the number on the scale is often the most obvious indicator of progress, it's far from the only one. In this chapter, we'll explore various methods to track your weight loss progress, ensuring that you have a comprehensive understanding of your body's changes and the improvements in your overall health.

Different methods to track weight loss progress

When embarking on a weight loss journey, it's natural to fixate on the number displayed on your bathroom scale. However, this singular focus can be misleading and potentially demotivating. Weight fluctuates daily due to various factors such as water retention, hormonal changes, and even the time of day you weigh yourself. Therefore, it's crucial to employ multiple tracking methods to get a more accurate picture of your progress.

One effective method is to weigh yourself consistently, but not obsessively. Choose a specific day and time each week, preferably in the morning after using the bathroom and before eating or drinking anything. This approach provides a more reliable trend over time, rather than getting caught up in daily fluctuations. Record these weekly weigh-ins in a journal or app to visualize your progress over the course of your 30-day challenge and beyond.

Another valuable tracking method is the use of a body fat caliper. This simple tool measures the thickness of skin folds at various points on your body, providing an estimate of your body fat percentage. While it requires some practice to use accurately, it can offer insights into changes in your body composition that the scale alone cannot reveal. As you lose fat and gain muscle through your new diet and exercise routine, you may find that your weight doesn't change dramatically, but your body fat percentage decreases – a clear sign of progress.

Bioelectrical impedance scales are another technology worth considering. These devices send a small, harmless electrical current through your body to estimate your body fat percentage, muscle mass, and water weight. While not as accurate as professional-grade equipment, they can provide a general trend of your body composition changes over time.

It's important to note that no single method is perfect, and each has its limitations. The key is to use a combination of these tracking methods to build a comprehensive picture of your progress. As Dr. Yoni Freedhoff, a renowned obesity medicine physician, states, "The scale is just one tool in the toolbox of health. It doesn't measure the quality of your diet, your fitness level, or your overall health and well-being."

Using body measurements and progress photos

While the scale and body fat measurements provide numerical data, they don't always capture the visible changes in your body shape and size. This is where body measurements and progress photos come into play, offering a visual and tangible representation of your weight loss journey.

Start by taking measurements of key areas of your body, including your chest, waist, hips, thighs, and arms. Use a flexible measuring tape and record these measurements weekly or bi-weekly. Often, you'll notice inches lost in these areas even when the scale hasn't budged, which can be incredibly motivating.

Progress photos are perhaps one of the most powerful tools in your tracking arsenal. Our brains are wired to recognize visual changes, but because we see ourselves every day, gradual changes can be hard to notice. By taking photos at regular intervals – ideally at the start of your journey and then every week or two – you create a visual timeline of your transformation.

When taking progress photos, consistency is key. Wear similar clothing (or lack thereof, if you're comfortable), use the same lighting and background, and take photos from the same angles each time. Front, side, and back views are typically most useful. These photos not only serve as motivation for you but can also be a powerful tool for accountability if you choose to share them with a support group or on social media.

Dr. John Berardi, a nutrition and exercise coach, emphasizes the importance of progress photos: "Photos and measurements are often more motivating than scale weight. They show people how their bodies are changing in ways that are meaningful to them."

Tracking non-scale victories

While physical changes are often the most noticeable, it's crucial not to overlook the myriad of other improvements that come with adopting a healthier lifestyle. These "non-scale victories" (NSVs) can be just as, if not more, important than the number on the scale.

One significant NSV to track is your energy levels. As you adopt healthier eating habits and increase your physical activity, you may notice that you have more energy throughout the day. You might find yourself needing less coffee to get through the afternoon slump, or having the energy to play with your children after a long day at work. Keep a journal to note these changes in your daily energy levels and overall mood.

Sleep quality is another important NSV to monitor. As you lose weight and improve your fitness, many people find that they sleep more soundly and wake up feeling more refreshed. You might notice that you fall asleep more easily, experience fewer night-time awakenings, or feel more alert in the mornings. These improvements in sleep quality can have far-reaching effects on your overall health and well-being.

Fitness improvements are also crucial NSVs to track. Perhaps when you started your 30-day challenge, you could only walk for 10 minutes before getting winded. As you progress, you might find yourself able to jog for 20 minutes or even run a full 5K. In strength training, you might notice that you can lift heavier weights or perform more repetitions of an exercise. These fitness gains are clear indicators of improved health and should be celebrated just as much as weight loss.

Another often overlooked NSV is the improvement in your relationship with food. As you learn more about nutrition and practice mindful eating, you may find that you no longer view food as the enemy or feel guilty after eating. Instead, you might develop a more balanced approach to nutrition, enjoying treats in moderation without derailing your progress. This shift in mentality is a significant victory that can lead to long-term success in maintaining a healthy weight.

Dr. Michelle May, author of "Eat What You Love, Love What You Eat," emphasizes the importance of these non-scale victories: "When you focus on the scale, you miss out on all the other amazing benefits of living a healthier lifestyle. By recognizing and celebrating these non-scale victories, you reinforce the positive changes you're making, making it more likely that you'll stick with your new habits long-term."

Adjusting goals and strategies based on progress

As you track your progress using various methods, it's important to regularly review and adjust your goals and strategies. Weight loss is not always a linear process, and what works in the beginning may not be as effective as you progress.

Start by reviewing your initial goals. Are they still realistic and aligned with your current progress? If you've surpassed your initial weight loss goal, it might be time to set new, more challenging targets. Conversely, if you're struggling to meet your original goals, it may be necessary to adjust them to more achievable levels. Remember, the goal is progress, not perfection.

Next, evaluate the effectiveness of your current strategies. If you've hit a plateau in your weight loss, it might be time to shake things up. This could involve changing your workout routine, adjusting your calorie intake, or trying new healthy recipes to prevent boredom with your meal plan. The key is to be flexible and willing to experiment to find what works best for your body.

It's also crucial to assess your emotional and mental state throughout your journey. Are you feeling motivated and energized, or are you struggling with feelings of deprivation or burnout? If it's the latter, it might be time to reassess your approach and find ways to make your new lifestyle more sustainable and enjoyable.

Dr. Traci Mann, a professor of psychology at the University of Minnesota and author of "Secrets From the Eating Lab," advises, "The most successful weight loss strategies are those that you can stick with long-term. If your current approach feels unsustainable, it's time to make adjustments."

As you near the end of your 30-day challenge, use the data you've collected to plan for the future. What strategies have been most effective for you? Which habits have you found easiest to maintain? Use this information to create a long-term plan that will help you maintain your progress and continue working towards your health goals.

Remember, tracking your progress is not just about monitoring weight loss. It's about gaining a deeper understanding of your body, celebrating your achievements, and continuously refining your approach to health and wellness. By employing a variety of tracking methods and regularly adjusting your strategies, you set yourself up for long-term success that goes far beyond the 30-day challenge.

As we move forward to the next chapter on overcoming plateaus, keep in mind that the skills you've developed in tracking your progress will be invaluable. Understanding the various ways your body changes and improves will help you push through challenges and continue making progress, even when the scale seems stubborn. The journey to a healthier you is a marathon, not a sprint, and the ability to track and celebrate your progress along the way will keep you motivated and moving forward.

Chapter 7: Overcoming Plateaus: Pushing Through Challenges

As we transition from our discussion on tracking progress, it's important to acknowledge that the weight loss journey is rarely a smooth, continuous descent. You've been diligently following your plan, seeing results, and feeling motivated. But suddenly, the numbers on the scale refuse to budge. Welcome to the dreaded weight loss plateau – a common and often frustrating challenge that nearly every individual on a weight loss journey encounters.

Understanding weight loss plateaus

Weight loss plateaus are a natural part of the body's adaptation process. When you first begin your weight loss journey, your body readily sheds excess pounds as it adjusts to the new calorie deficit and increased physical activity. However, as you continue to lose weight, your body's metabolism naturally slows down. This is because a smaller body requires fewer calories to maintain its functions.

Dr. David Ludwig, a professor of nutrition at Harvard School of Public Health, explains this phenomenon: "As we lose weight, the body fights back in multiple ways, making it more and more difficult to continue losing weight at the same rate. It's not a failure of willpower; it's biology." This biological response is rooted in our evolutionary past, where the body's primary goal was to prevent starvation during times of food scarcity.

Furthermore, as you lose fat, you may also be gaining muscle, especially if you've incorporated strength training into your routine. Muscle tissue is denser than fat, which means that even though your body composition is improving, the number on the scale might not reflect these positive changes.

It's crucial to understand that plateaus are not indicative of failure. They are a sign that your body is adjusting to your new lifestyle and that it's time to reassess and possibly modify your approach. Recognizing this can help alleviate the frustration and disappointment that often accompanies a plateau, allowing you to approach the challenge with a more positive and proactive mindset.

Strategies to break through stagnation

Breaking through a weight loss plateau requires a multi-faceted approach. The key is to shake things up and challenge your body in new ways. Here are several strategies that can help you overcome this hurdle:

Reassess your calorie intake: As you've lost weight, your body now requires fewer calories to function. It's time to recalculate your daily calorie needs based on your current weight. You may need to further reduce your calorie intake, but be cautious not to drop too low, as this can be counterproductive and potentially harmful.

Increase the intensity of your workouts: Your body becomes more efficient at performing exercises it's used to, which means it burns fewer calories doing the same activities. Try incorporating high-intensity interval training (HIIT) into your routine. HIIT has been shown to be particularly effective at boosting metabolism and burning fat. A study published in the Journal of Obesity found that HIIT was more effective at reducing body fat compared to traditional steady-state cardio.

Mix up your exercise routine: Introduce new types of exercises to challenge your body in different ways. If you've been focusing on cardio, add strength training to your regimen. If you've been lifting weights, try incorporating yoga or Pilates to improve flexibility and engage different muscle groups.

Focus on protein intake: Increasing your protein consumption can help preserve muscle mass during weight loss and boost your metabolism. A study published in the American Journal of Clinical Nutrition found that a high-protein diet was more effective at preserving lean body mass during weight loss compared to a standard-protein diet.

Get enough sleep: Lack of sleep can disrupt hormones that regulate hunger and metabolism. Aim for 7-9 hours of quality sleep each night. A study in the Annals of Internal Medicine showed that insufficient sleep can reduce the amount of weight lost from fat by 55% and increase the loss of fat-free body mass.

Manage stress: Chronic stress can lead to elevated cortisol levels, which can interfere with weight loss. Incorporate stress-reduction techniques such as meditation, deep breathing exercises, or regular massages into your routine.

Try intermittent fasting: Some individuals find success with intermittent fasting, which involves cycling between periods of eating and fasting. While not suitable for everyone, it can be an effective way to break through a plateau for some. Always consult with a healthcare professional before making significant changes to your eating patterns.

Importance of consistency and patience

When faced with a plateau, it's tempting to make drastic changes or give up entirely. However, consistency and patience are your most powerful allies in overcoming this challenge. Remember that weight loss is not always linear, and fluctuations are normal.

Dr. Yoni Freedhoff, medical director of the Bariatric Medical Institute in Ottawa, emphasizes the importance of consistency: "The most important habit you can cultivate is the habit of perseverance. Weight loss is a lifelong journey, not a sprint to a finish line."

Maintain your healthy habits even when the scale isn't moving. Continue to eat nutritious foods, stay hydrated, exercise regularly, and get adequate sleep. These behaviors are beneficial for your overall health, regardless of weight loss.

It's also crucial to practice self-compassion during this time. Negative self-talk and frustration can lead to stress eating or abandoning healthy habits altogether. Instead, view the plateau as a normal part of the process and an opportunity to refine your approach.

Keep in mind that weight loss often occurs in stages. You might experience periods of rapid loss followed by plateaus. This pattern is often referred to as the "whoosh effect," where your body seems to resist weight loss for a period before suddenly dropping several pounds at once.

Adjusting nutrition and exercise plans

Breaking through a plateau often requires fine-tuning your nutrition and exercise plans. Here are some specific adjustments you can consider:

Nutrition adjustments:

Re-evaluate your portion sizes: Even if you're eating healthy foods, portion creep can occur over time. Use measuring tools or a food scale to ensure you're not unconsciously increasing your portions.

Increase your fiber intake: Fiber-rich foods can help you feel fuller for longer and may aid in weight loss. Aim for at least 25-30 grams of fiber per day from sources like vegetables, fruits, whole grains, and legumes.

Experiment with meal timing: Some people find success with eating smaller, more frequent meals throughout the day, while others do better with larger, less frequent meals. Experiment to find what works best for your body and lifestyle.

Stay hydrated: Sometimes, thirst can be mistaken for hunger. Ensure you're drinking enough water throughout the day. A study in the Journal of Clinical Endocrinology and Metabolism found that drinking 500ml of water increased metabolic rate by 30% in both men and women.

Exercise adjustments:

Progressive overload: Gradually increase the weight, frequency, or number of repetitions in your strength training routine. This challenges your muscles and can help boost your metabolism.

Try new activities: If you've been sticking to the same exercise routine, your body may have adapted. Introduce new activities like swimming, cycling, or dance classes to challenge your body in different ways.

Non-exercise activity thermogenesis (NEAT): Increase your overall daily movement outside of structured exercise. Take the stairs instead of the elevator, park further away from your destination, or do some light stretching during TV commercials.

Active recovery: On your rest days, engage in light activities like yoga or walking to keep your body moving without overexerting yourself.

Remember, the key to breaking through a plateau is to make small, sustainable changes rather than drastic overhauls. Dr. Holly Wyatt, a professor of medicine at the University of Colorado, advises: "The goal is to find a way of eating and exercising that you can stick with for the long haul. It's not about quick fixes; it's about lifestyle change."

As you implement these strategies, be patient with yourself and your body. It may take some time to see results, but persistence is key. Keep track of your efforts and any changes you experience, not just in weight but also in how you feel, your energy levels, and your overall well-being.

Breaking through a weight loss plateau can be challenging, but it's an opportunity for growth and refinement of your health journey. By understanding the science behind plateaus, implementing targeted strategies, maintaining consistency, and making thoughtful adjustments to your plan, you can overcome this obstacle and continue progressing towards your goals.

As we move forward, it's important to recognize that the support of others can play a crucial role in helping you navigate these challenges. In the next chapter, we'll explore how to build and leverage a support network to enhance your weight loss journey, providing you with the encouragement and accountability needed to push through plateaus and other obstacles you may encounter along the way.

Chapter 8: Social Support: Leveraging Relationships for Success

As we transition from the challenges of overcoming plateaus, we now turn our attention to an often overlooked yet crucial aspect of successful weight loss: social support. The journey to a healthier you doesn't have to be a solitary one. In fact, leveraging your relationships and building a strong support network can significantly enhance your chances of achieving and maintaining your weight loss goals.

Building a support network is not just about having cheerleaders in your corner; it's about creating an environment that nurtures your new healthy lifestyle. This network can include family members, friends, colleagues, or even online communities of like-minded individuals. The key is to surround yourself with people who understand your goals and are willing to support you through the ups and downs of your weight loss journey.

One of the most effective ways to build a support network is to be open about your goals and challenges. Share your aspirations with those close to you, explaining why this journey is important to you. You might be surprised by how many people are willing to offer encouragement and practical support. As Dr. Robert Cialdini, a renowned psychologist, notes in his book "Influence: The Psychology of Persuasion," "Public commitments tend to be lasting commitments." By sharing your goals, you're not only gaining support but also creating a sense of accountability.

Consider involving your family members in your new healthy lifestyle. This could mean cooking nutritious meals together, going for walks after dinner, or even having friendly competitions to see who can reach their daily step goal. By making health a family affair, you're not only building a support system but also positively influencing the habits of those around you.

Friends can also play a crucial role in your support network. Look for workout buddies or meal prep partners among your friends. Having someone to exercise with not only makes the activity more enjoyable but also increases your commitment. A study published in the Journal of Social Sciences found that people tend to gravitate towards the exercise behaviors of those around them. So, surrounding yourself with active friends can naturally boost your own activity levels.

However, building a support network isn't always smooth sailing. You may encounter individuals who, intentionally or not, undermine your efforts. These could be friends who constantly pressure you to indulge in unhealthy foods or family members who dismiss your goals. Navigating these social situations requires tact and assertiveness.

When faced with unsupportive individuals, it's important to communicate clearly and firmly about your goals and boundaries. Explain that while you value their company, you're committed to your health journey. You might say something like, "I appreciate the offer, but I'm focusing on my health right now. I'd love to spend time with you in a way that aligns with my goals. How about we go for a walk together instead?"

Remember, you don't need to apologize for prioritizing your health. As motivational speaker Jim Rohn famously said, "You are the average of the five people you spend the most time with." If certain relationships consistently undermine your efforts, it may be necessary to reevaluate how much time and energy you invest in them.

Navigating social situations and dining out can be particularly challenging when you're trying to lose weight. However, with the right strategies, you can maintain your social life without derailing your progress. When dining out, review the menu in advance if possible and decide on a healthy option before you arrive. This reduces the likelihood of making impulsive choices based on what others are ordering.

Don't be afraid to make special requests at restaurants. Most establishments are happy to accommodate dietary needs. You could ask for dressings on the side, vegetables instead of fries, or grilled options instead of fried. Remember, you're not being difficult; you're taking care of your health.

When attending social gatherings, consider bringing a healthy dish to share. This ensures you have at least one option that aligns with your goals and allows you to introduce others to tasty, nutritious alternatives. You might be surprised by how many people appreciate having a healthier option available.

In today's digital age, social support extends beyond in-person interactions. Social media and mobile apps can be powerful tools for motivation and accountability. Platforms like Instagram and Facebook host numerous weight loss and fitness communities where you can connect with others on similar journeys, share experiences, and gain inspiration.

Consider joining online forums or groups dedicated to healthy living. These communities can provide a wealth of information, from recipe ideas to workout tips. They also offer a space to share your struggles and triumphs with people who understand exactly what you're going through. As social psychologist Dr. Stephen Franzoi points out, "Sharing personal experiences with others who have gone through similar situations can be incredibly validating and motivating."

Mobile apps can also play a significant role in your support network. Many weight loss and fitness apps include social features that allow you to connect with friends or join challenges. These features tap into the power of friendly competition and social accountability to keep you motivated. For example, you might join a step challenge with colleagues or share your workout achievements with friends through the app.

However, it's important to use social media and apps mindfully. While they can be great sources of support and motivation, they can also lead to unhealthy comparisons or unrealistic expectations. Remember that everyone's journey is unique, and what works for one person may not work for another. Use these platforms as tools for inspiration and connection, not as measuring sticks for your own progress.

One often overlooked aspect of social support is becoming a source of support for others. As you progress in your journey, consider mentoring someone who's just starting out. Sharing your experiences and offering encouragement to others can reinforce your own commitment to a healthy lifestyle. It's a powerful reminder of how far you've come and can provide renewed motivation when you face challenges.

Building and leveraging a strong support network is not a one-time task but an ongoing process. As you progress in your weight loss journey, your needs may change, and so might your support network. Be open to forming new connections and don't be afraid to distance yourself from relationships that no longer serve your goals.

Remember, seeking support is not a sign of weakness but a strategy for success. Even professional athletes have coaches and support teams to help them perform at their best. By building a robust support network, you're giving yourself the best possible chance of achieving and maintaining your weight loss goals.

As we conclude this chapter on social support, it's clear that the relationships we cultivate can have a profound impact on our weight loss journey. From family and friends to online communities, each component of your support network plays a unique role in your success. As we move forward, we'll explore how to maintain the momentum you've built over these 30 days and turn your short-term efforts into long-lasting lifestyle changes. The next chapter will delve into strategies for staying motivated in the long run, ensuring that your weight loss journey doesn't end when the challenge does.

Chapter 9: Maintaining Momentum: Staying Motivated in the Long Run

As we approach the final stages of our 30-day weight loss challenge, it's crucial to shift our focus towards maintaining the momentum we've built. The journey doesn't end here; in fact, this is where the real test begins. Sustaining weight loss and continuing to progress towards our health goals requires a different mindset and approach than the initial push. In this chapter, we'll explore strategies to keep you motivated, set new goals, celebrate your achievements, and handle the inevitable setbacks that come with any long-term lifestyle change.

Setting new goals after the 30-day challenge is an essential step in maintaining your momentum. The completion of the challenge marks a significant milestone, but it's just the beginning of your lifelong journey towards health and wellness. As you look beyond the 30 days, it's time to reassess your progress and determine what you want to achieve next. This process of goal-setting should be thoughtful and deliberate, taking into account both your achievements so far and your long-term aspirations.

Start by reflecting on your initial goals for the challenge. Did you meet them? Exceed them? Or perhaps you fell short in some areas? Regardless of the outcome, use this information to inform your next set of goals. If you successfully lost the weight you aimed for, perhaps your next goal could be to increase your strength or improve your endurance. If you struggled with consistency in your workout routine, maybe your next goal could be to establish a regular exercise habit, aiming for a specific number of workouts per week.

Remember, effective goal-setting follows the SMART criteria: Specific, Measurable, Achievable, Relevant, and Time-bound. Instead of a vague goal like "get fitter," try something like "run a 5K race in under 30 minutes within the next three months." This goal is specific (run a 5K), measurable (under 30 minutes), achievable (assuming you've been building your fitness during the challenge), relevant to your overall health journey, and time-bound (within the next three months).

It's also important to set a mix of short-term and long-term goals. Short-term goals provide immediate targets to work towards and help maintain motivation, while long-term goals give you a broader vision to aspire to. For example, a short-term goal might be to try a new healthy recipe each week for the next month, while a long-term goal could be to compete in a half-marathon by the end of the year.

As you continue on your health journey, don't forget to celebrate your achievements and milestones along the way. Too often, we focus solely on the end goal and forget to acknowledge the progress we've made. Celebrating your successes, no matter how small, is crucial for maintaining motivation and building a positive association with your healthy habits.

These celebrations don't have to be grand gestures or involve breaking your healthy habits. In fact, the best celebrations reinforce your new lifestyle. For example, if you've successfully stuck to your workout routine for a month, you might treat yourself to a new piece of workout gear or a massage to help with muscle recovery. If you've consistently met your nutrition goals, perhaps you could splurge on a high-quality ingredient to use in a healthy gourmet meal you prepare at home.

Remember to celebrate non-scale victories as well. Did your energy levels improve? Are you sleeping better? Can you now easily climb the stairs without getting winded? These are all significant achievements that deserve recognition. Keep a journal to track these improvements – it can serve as a powerful motivator when you're feeling discouraged.

Sharing your achievements with your support network can also be a form of celebration. Not only does it allow you to bask in your success, but it can also inspire and motivate others. As fitness expert Jillian Michaels once said, "Whenever you get to a place in your life where you feel proud of yourself, share it with people. It can inspire others to do the same and create a positive ripple effect."

Developing a long-term healthy lifestyle mindset is perhaps the most crucial aspect of maintaining momentum after the 30-day challenge. This involves shifting your perspective from seeing your new habits as a temporary "diet" or "exercise program" to viewing them as an integral part of your lifestyle.

This mindset shift doesn't happen overnight. It requires consistent effort and a conscious decision to prioritize your health every day. Start by re-framing how you think about your choices. Instead of saying, "I can't eat that because I'm on a diet," try, "I choose not to eat that because it doesn't align with my health goals." This simple change in language emphasizes that you're in control of your choices and that these choices are part of a broader lifestyle, not a restrictive short-term plan.

Another key aspect of developing a long-term mindset is finding joy in your new habits. If you view healthy eating and exercise as punishment or deprivation, you're unlikely to stick with them in the long run. Instead, focus on the positive aspects of your new lifestyle. Maybe you've discovered a love for cooking nutritious meals, or perhaps you've found that your morning jog is a peaceful time for self-reflection. Lean into these positive experiences and let them fuel your motivation.

It's also important to remain flexible and adaptable in your approach. Life is unpredictable, and there will be times when sticking to your usual routine is challenging. Instead of seeing these as failures, view them as opportunities to problem-solve and adapt. Maybe you can't make it to the gym due to a busy work schedule – that's okay. Can you do a quick home workout instead? Or perhaps go for a brisk walk during your lunch break? This adaptability is key to maintaining a healthy lifestyle in the face of life's inevitable curveballs.

Handling setbacks and getting back on track is an essential skill for long-term success. No matter how committed you are to your goals, there will be times when you slip up or face challenges that derail your progress temporarily. The key is not to let these setbacks turn into complete derailments.

First and foremost, it's crucial to approach setbacks with self-compassion. Beating yourself up over a missed workout or an indulgent meal is counterproductive and can lead to a negative spiral. Instead, acknowledge the setback without judgment, and then focus on getting back on track.

As fitness guru Richard Simmons once said, "You can't go back and change the beginning, but you can start where you are and change the ending." This quote encapsulates the mindset needed to overcome setbacks. Instead of dwelling on what went wrong, focus on what you can do right now to get back on track.

One effective strategy for handling setbacks is to have a pre-planned "reset" routine. This could be a specific meal plan for the day after an indulgence, or a favorite workout that helps you feel strong and capable. Having this plan in place takes the guesswork out of getting back on track and provides a clear path forward.

It's also helpful to analyze your setbacks for valuable lessons. Was there a particular trigger that led to overeating? Did a change in your schedule make it difficult to fit in your usual workout? Understanding these factors can help you develop strategies to prevent similar setbacks in the future or handle them more effectively when they do occur.

Remember, progress is not linear. There will be ups and downs, but it's the overall trend that matters. As long as you're moving in the right direction most of the time, you're on the path to success.

As we conclude this chapter on maintaining momentum, it's important to recognize that the journey you've embarked on is a lifelong one. The habits and mindset you've developed during this 30-day challenge are the foundation for a healthier, happier life. By setting new goals, celebrating your achievements, developing a long-term healthy lifestyle mindset, and learning to handle setbacks effectively, you're well-equipped to continue your progress beyond this challenge.

In the next and final chapter, we'll explore how to transition from active weight loss to weight maintenance, further integrate your new healthy habits into your daily life, continue challenging yourself with new fitness goals, and even inspire others with your success story. Remember, every step you take towards a healthier lifestyle, no matter how small, is a victory worth celebrating. Keep moving forward, stay committed to your goals, and trust in the process. Your journey to a healthier you is just beginning.

Chapter 10: Beyond 30 Days: Sustaining Your New Healthy Lifestyle

As we reach the culmination of our 30-day weight loss challenge, it's important to recognize that this is not the end, but rather the beginning of a new chapter in your life. The journey you've embarked upon over the past month has equipped you with valuable tools, insights, and habits that can serve as the foundation for a sustainable, healthy lifestyle. In this final chapter, we'll explore how to transition from the structured 30-day program to a long-term approach that will help you maintain your weight loss and continue to thrive in your newfound health and wellness.

Transitioning from weight loss to weight maintenance

The shift from active weight loss to weight maintenance is a crucial phase that many people struggle with. It's essential to understand that the strategies that helped you lose weight may need to be adjusted to help you maintain your new weight. As you transition, you'll need to recalibrate your calorie intake and exercise routine to find the right balance that allows you to maintain your weight without feeling deprived or overworked.

One of the first steps in this transition is to gradually increase your calorie intake. During your weight loss phase, you likely created a calorie deficit to shed pounds. Now, you'll need to find your maintenance calorie level – the number of calories that allows you to maintain your current weight. This process may involve some trial and error, and it's important to be patient with yourself as you find the right balance.

Dr. David Katz, founding director of Yale University's Prevention Research Center, emphasizes the importance of this transition: "The key to successful weight maintenance is to make sustainable changes. It's not about dieting forever; it's about finding a way of eating and living that you can stick with for the long haul."

In addition to adjusting your calorie intake, you'll need to continue with regular physical activity. The Centers for Disease Control and Prevention (CDC) recommends at least 150 minutes of moderate-intensity aerobic activity or 75 minutes of vigorous-intensity aerobic activity per week for adults, along with muscle-strengthening activities at least twice a week. This level of activity not only helps with weight maintenance but also provides numerous other health benefits.

It's also crucial to continue monitoring your weight and body composition regularly. While daily weigh-ins may not be necessary, checking your weight once a week or every two weeks can help you stay on track and catch any potential weight regain early. Remember that some fluctuations are normal, and it's the overall trend that matters most.

As you transition, be prepared for potential challenges. Your body may try to regain the lost weight, a phenomenon known as "adaptive thermogenesis." This is why it's crucial to remain vigilant and committed to your healthy habits. Dr. Michael Roizen, Chief Wellness Officer at the Cleveland Clinic, notes, "Your body will fight to regain the weight. It's not a personal failure; it's biology. The key is to be aware of this tendency and to have strategies in place to combat it."

Incorporating new healthy habits into daily life

The 30-day challenge has introduced you to a variety of healthy habits. Now, the goal is to weave these habits seamlessly into the fabric of your daily life. This process of habit formation is critical for long-term success. According to research by Phillippa Lally and her colleagues at University

College London, it takes an average of 66 days for a new behavior to become automatic. This underscores the importance of consistency and patience as you work to solidify your new healthy lifestyle.

One effective strategy for incorporating healthy habits is to link them to existing routines. For example, if you've developed the habit of drinking a glass of water first thing in the morning during the challenge, you can reinforce this by always placing a glass of water on your nightstand before bed. This visual cue will remind you to hydrate as soon as you wake up.

Meal planning and preparation, which you likely practiced during the challenge, should continue to be a cornerstone of your healthy lifestyle. By dedicating time each week to plan and prepare meals, you can ensure that you always have nutritious options on hand, reducing the likelihood of impulsive, unhealthy food choices. Consider experimenting with new healthy recipes to keep your meals interesting and varied.

Physical activity should remain a priority in your daily life. If you've found exercises or activities that you enjoy, make them a regular part of your schedule. If you're struggling to find time for formal workouts, look for ways to incorporate more movement into your daily routine. This could include taking the stairs instead of the elevator, walking or biking for short errands, or even standing up and stretching every hour if you have a sedentary job.

Mindful eating practices should also continue beyond the 30-day challenge. Pay attention to your hunger and fullness cues, eat slowly, and savor your meals. These habits can help prevent overeating and promote a healthier relationship with food. Dr. Susan Albers, a psychologist and mindful eating expert, advises, "Mindful eating isn't about being perfect, it's about being present. When you eat mindfully, you're more likely to make choices that nourish your body and satisfy your hunger."

Stress management techniques that you've learned during the challenge should become part of your daily routine. Whether it's meditation, deep breathing exercises, yoga, or any other stress-reduction method that works for you, make time for these practices regularly. Managing stress is crucial not only for weight maintenance but also for overall health and well-being.

Adequate sleep should remain a priority in your new lifestyle. Aim for 7-9 hours of quality sleep each night. Maintain a consistent sleep schedule, create a relaxing bedtime routine, and ensure your sleep environment is conducive to rest. Dr. Matthew Walker, Professor of Neuroscience and Psychology at the University of California, Berkeley, emphasizes, "Sleep is the single most effective thing we can do to reset our brain and body health each day."

Remember that incorporating these habits into your daily life is an ongoing process. Be patient with yourself and celebrate the small victories along the way. Each day that you make healthy choices is a step towards cementing these habits as an integral part of your lifestyle.

Continuing to challenge yourself with fitness goals

While maintaining your weight is a significant achievement, it's important to continue setting new goals to keep yourself motivated and to further improve your health and fitness. These goals can help prevent complacency and provide a sense of purpose and direction in your fitness journey.

One approach is to set performance-based goals rather than solely focusing on weight. These could include improving your strength, endurance, flexibility, or overall fitness level. For example, you might aim to run a 5K race, master a challenging yoga pose, or increase the amount of weight you can lift in a particular exercise.

Dr. Michelle Segar, director of the University of Michigan's Sport, Health, and Activity Research and Policy Center, suggests, "Setting goals that focus on immediate positive payoffs, like how exercise makes you feel energized or reduces stress, can be more motivating than distant goals like preventing heart disease."

Consider trying new forms of exercise or physical activities. This not only challenges your body in different ways but also keeps your fitness routine fresh and exciting. You might explore activities like rock climbing, dance classes, martial arts, or team sports. The variety can help prevent boredom and provide a more well-rounded fitness experience.

High-Intensity Interval Training (HIIT) can be an excellent addition to your fitness routine. HIIT workouts involve short bursts of intense exercise followed by periods of rest or lower-intensity activity. These workouts are efficient, effective for burning calories, and can help improve cardiovascular health. However, it's important to gradually incorporate HIIT into your routine and to listen to your body to avoid overtraining.

Strength training should continue to be a key component of your fitness regimen. As you progress, you can challenge yourself by increasing weights, trying more complex exercises, or incorporating techniques like supersets or drop sets. Remember to maintain proper form and technique as you advance to prevent injuries.

Setting specific, measurable, achievable, relevant, and time-bound (SMART) goals can help you stay focused and motivated. For example, instead of a vague goal like "get stronger," you might aim to "increase my squat weight by 20 pounds in the next three months." This specific goal gives you a clear target to work towards and a timeline for achieving it.

Consider participating in fitness challenges or events. This could be a local 10K run, a charity bike ride, or a community fitness challenge. Having a specific event to prepare for can provide structure to your training and a sense of accomplishment when you complete it.

Remember that as you continue to challenge yourself, it's crucial to listen to your body and allow for adequate rest and recovery. Overtraining can lead to burnout, decreased performance, and increased risk of injury. Incorporate rest days into your routine and pay attention to signs that your body needs more recovery time.

Dr. Jordan Metzl, a sports medicine physician at Hospital for Special Surgery in New York City, advises, "The key to long-term fitness success is finding a balance between pushing yourself and allowing for recovery. It's during rest periods that your body adapts and becomes stronger."

Sharing your success and inspiring others

As you continue your journey beyond the 30-day challenge, you have a unique opportunity to inspire and motivate others who may be at the beginning of their own health and fitness journeys. Sharing your experiences, challenges, and successes can not only help others but also reinforce your own commitment to a healthy lifestyle.

One way to share your story is through social media platforms. You can post about your progress, share healthy recipes you've discovered, or demonstrate exercises you've found effective. However, it's important to do this in a way that's authentic and respectful of others' journeys. Focus on sharing your personal experiences rather than giving unsolicited advice.

Consider starting a blog or vlog to document your ongoing journey. This can serve as a personal record of your progress and provide inspiration to others. It can also help keep you accountable as you continue to pursue your health and fitness goals.

Participating in online or in-person support groups can be another way to share your experiences and learn from others. These groups can provide a sense of community and mutual support, which can be invaluable in maintaining long-term motivation.

If you feel comfortable, you might consider becoming a mentor to someone who is just starting their weight loss journey. Sharing your insights and offering support can be incredibly rewarding and can help reinforce your own healthy habits.

Remember that everyone's journey is unique, and what worked for you may not work for everyone. When sharing your experiences, emphasize the importance of finding an approach that is sustainable and enjoyable for each individual.

Dr. Yoni Freedhoff, medical director of the Bariatric Medical Institute in Ottawa, suggests, "The best diet is the one you don't know you're on. By sharing how you've made healthy living a natural part of your life, you can inspire others to find their own sustainable path."

As you share your success, be prepared for questions and even skepticism from others. Use these interactions as opportunities to educate and inspire, but also remember that you're not responsible for others' choices or behaviors.

Lastly, don't forget to celebrate your own ongoing success. Recognize the hard work and dedication that has brought you to this point, and continue to acknowledge your achievements, both big and small. Your journey is a testament to the power of commitment and perseverance, and by living your best, healthiest life, you become a beacon of inspiration to others.

As we conclude this chapter and this book, remember that the end of the 30-day challenge is just the beginning of your lifelong journey towards health and wellness. The habits you've developed, the knowledge you've gained, and the resilience you've built will serve you well as you continue to grow and thrive. Embrace the challenges ahead, celebrate your successes, and never stop striving for your best, healthiest self. Your 30-day challenge may be complete, but your incredible journey of health and self-discovery is just beginning.

Conclusion:

As we reach the end of our 30-day journey, it's clear that weight loss is about more than just shedding pounds. It's a holistic process that involves nutrition, exercise, sleep, stress management, and social support. Throughout this book, we've explored how small, consistent changes in these areas can lead to significant results. From understanding macronutrients to developing smart eating habits, from incorporating regular exercise to managing stress, each step has been designed to help you achieve your weight loss goals.

The importance of tracking progress and overcoming plateaus cannot be overstated. By measuring success beyond the scale and learning to push through challenges, you've developed resilience and adaptability. These skills will serve you well not just in your weight loss journey, but in all aspects of life. Remember, progress isn't always linear, and setbacks are a normal part of any transformative process.

Your 30-day challenge may be coming to an end, but your journey towards a healthier lifestyle is just beginning. The habits and knowledge you've gained over the past month form a solid foundation for long-term success. As you transition from active weight loss to weight maintenance, continue to set new goals, celebrate your achievements, and inspire others with your progress.

The most crucial takeaway from this experience is the development of a sustainable, healthy lifestyle. Weight loss isn't about quick fixes or extreme measures; it's about making lasting changes that improve your overall well-being. By focusing on nourishing your body, staying active, managing stress, and surrounding yourself with support, you've created a blueprint for lifelong health and happiness.

As you move forward, remember that your journey is unique. What works for one person may not work for another, and that's okay. The key is to stay committed to your health goals while being flexible and kind to yourself. Continue to challenge yourself, learn from setbacks, and celebrate every victory, no matter how small. Your transformation over these 30 days is just the beginning of a new, healthier you.